Water, Dehydration and Computer Use:

Learn How to Protect Yourself

By

Adetutu Ijose

Published By:

Jointheirs Publishing

JP

Water, Dehydration and Computer Use: Learn How to Protect Yourself

Jointheirs Publishing
Jointheirs Activities Incorporated
www.jointheirspublishing.com

ISBN – 1-46363-805-1

EAN – 978-1-46363-805-4

Printed in the United States of America

Water, Dehydration and Computer Use:

Learn How to Protect Yourself

An Important Caution

The advice given in *Water Dehydration and Computer Use* is based on an understanding of the effects of computer use on human health and behavior gained when I suffered life threatening consequences of computer use that could not be effectively diagnosed or treated by conventional medical science.

I was only able to get an understanding of the problem and identify the solution by studying and gaining an understanding of the human code of existence from studying the System of Nature and human machine user manual we call the Bible or Scriptures.

It tells us that the earth was created in water and the water had to break in order to bring forth the earth, as we know it. This is much like the way humans are born. The fetus lives in a sack of water that is broken before the child is born and exposed into the atmosphere of the earth.

Unbeknown to many, computer use is guilty of dehydrating the human body.

This book tells us why and how this occurs and suggests practical solutions to the problem

As in all my other books, I urge the reader to read the entire book and study it carefully.

It is essential that any decision you make be discussed with your physician and if you are a not yet an adult your parents or any other person of authority in your life before proceeding.

This book is not meant to replace the advice of parents or the service of a health care provider who knows you personally.

An essential element of taking responsibility for your life and health is a regular medical checkup working in partnership with medical professionals and counselors and if you are not yet an adult, having a good relationship with your parents and other persons in authority over you.

If you are under treatment for any computer use induced health condition or if you suspect you might need such care, you must discuss any insight you gain from this book with your doctor before starting.

Again, please read the entire book carefully and help yourself and all you know.

You can be a long-term computer user without self-destroying but you must first acknowledge the need to do something.

All the solutions are natural, cheap and do not involve medication. In fact medicine is stressful to the body and one that is already weakened from the health effects of computer use should not be medicated. That will increase the stress and start a new problems involving unnecessary costs that could bankrupt individuals and societally as a nation and even globally.

We therefore need to change the way we have been looking at this issue if we want to remain a healthy prosperous population on earth.

One thing though, you must not self diagnose just look for a doctor who is ready to use other measures apart from medication as you will need close monitoring and some tests to identify what is depleted or missing in your body's system as a result of your computer use. These tests do not show everything but are a good starting point.

Computers are here to stay and can never be as safe as claimed. The computer use environment for example makes us look directly at a source of light to read, which is contrary to our natural way of never looking directly at the sun (our natural source of reading light).

Table of Contents

Chapter 1
Water, Water, Water and the Beginning

One of the major things that we all learn in school that we experience daily is the fact that over 60% of the human body is made of water and that without water it is impossible to stay alive.

We all hear that everyday we should drink a glass of water first thing every morning to aid our body in passing out fecal waste.

According to the United States Geological Survey (USGS) Water Science School [1-1] "Up to 60% of the human body is water, the brain is composed of 70% water, and the lungs are nearly 90% water.

Lean muscle tissue contains about 75% water by weight, as is the brain; body fat contains 10% water and bone has 22% water. About 83% of our blood is water, which helps digest our food, transport waste, and control body temperature.

Each day humans must replace 2.4 litres of water, some through drinking and the rest taken by the body from the foods eaten."

It also says that" The carbohydrates and proteins that our bodies use as food are metabolized and transported by water in the bloodstream. No less important is the ability of water to transport waste material out of our bodies".

We humans need both external and internal hydration like everything else with life on planet earth. We also need our environment to be hydrated. Moisture is required for existence on earth. Even the desert air is hydrated. It is just that the level of hydration is less than in other places due to lack of rivers, lakes and other bodies of water in abundant numbers as is available everywhere else.

Air however moves around in the form of wind mixing dry air with moisture laden air from other parts of the earth to enable desert air maintain the level of moisture content required to maintain the moisture balance on the earth.

In fact drying up is one of the processes that takes place as loss of life commences and it progresses until final decay sets in and the object or person ceases to exist or be visible as it totally dries up and decomposes back into the dust of the earth i.e. back to the dust from where it came as we are told in the user manual we call the Bible or Scriptures.

The presence of water on the earth is in fact one of the first things we are told about in the manual underscoring the importance of water.

It tells us as we read in the "Important Caution", that the earth was born in it much like humans are born. The fetus lives in a sack of water that is broken before the child is born and exposed into the atmosphere of the earth.

It seems the body must be conditioned and the skin made to learn to operate in a hydrated system - absorb water and learn to absorb the light fields it needs to operate through water before the human body can dwell on earth. It is not a coincidence that water is the medium through which a lot of our research and innovation is carried out.

This shows us that the natural environmental coded requirement of starting in a water-based environment cannot be violated.

The manual tells us, that is how the earth began. It was hidden in water in darkness

This is the same way the fetus is encased in a sack of water in the womb away from direct light for 9 months during which the development to baby process occurs.

We are not told how long the earth was incubated in water but after some time light was brought in to begin the process of the life of the earth.

This is replicated in human birth and development. We will read more of this in chapter 7 "The summary" when we tie everything in prior chapters together to provide the grand picture of water, dehydration and computer use.

As we have read, the manual tells us the earth was created surrounded by water and was incubated in water in darkness and unseen until the time of its revelation when external light was provided and the water split into two to reveal what had been incubating in it.

This is much like what happens whenever new life is being brought forth into the earth whether of humans or animals.

They are always incubated in water and when they are ready to be exposed to external light and their bodies have learned how to self hydrate or their self hydrating function is fully operational and they can receive hydration in an environment with direct exposure to sunlight.

They have grown to the point where they cannot continue to grow without more light, the water breaks and they are born.

Therefore, without being incubated in water nothing can be born unto the earth.

Consequently, anything that affects the supply of moisture to hydrate the human body or that affects the availability of moisture containing environment in which to live and exist affects the auto hydration process of the human body.

This is dangerous to humans.

The manual also tells us that he earth when it was created was null and void and did not exist as a planet with mountains and hills, vegetation, humans, animals and so on as we know it today but was in water and indiscernible.

Even so the egg and sperm hidden in the water in the mother's womb and not discernible directly by the human eye, fuses to become the fetus that grows to be a human. The human body is hidden in the fetus in the womb and grows to become a baby who when born grows to become someone who can walk around on two feet.

If the mother's womb loses the water and becomes dry for some reason, the fetus would probably not survive and the mother may also lose her life.

Such is the importance of water and hydration for human life right from its beginning and throughout life.

Finally, the manual tells us that life is light and consequently it needs physical water to pass through, operate and dwell in us on the physiological physical level.

Chapter 2
Some facts about water

The USGS [1-1] says that according to Dr. Jeffrey Utz, Neuroscience, pediatrics, Allegheny University, "different people have different percentages of their bodies made up of water.

Babies have the most, being born at about 78%. By one year of age, that amount drops to about 65%. In adult men, about 60% of their bodies are water. However, fat tissue does not have as much water as lean tissue.

In adult women, fat makes up more of the body than men, so they have about 55% of their bodies made of water.

Thus babies and kids have more water (as a percentage) than adults.

Women have less water than men (as a percentage). People with more fatty tissue have less water than people with less fatty tissue (as a percentage)'.

This may be why women get more easily dehyrated.

According to the Better Health Channel BHC), a service fully funded by the State Government of Victoria (Australia). In their article on water [2-1],

"The human body can last weeks without food, but only days without water. The body is made up of 55–75 per cent water. Water forms the basis of blood, digestive juices, urine and perspiration and is contained in lean muscle, fat and bones.

As the body can't store water, it needs fresh supplies every day to make up for losses from lungs, skin, urine and fecal waste.

The article lists factors that determine the amount of water needed – body metabolism, the weather, the kind of food eaten and individual activity levels.

Factors that affect Internal body water supply:
1. Body water is higher in men than in women and falls in both with age. Most mature adults lose about 2.5–3 liters of water per day. Water loss may be more in hot weather and with prolonged exercise.

2. Elderly people lose about two liters per day

3. An air traveler can lose approximately 1.5 liters of water during a three-hour flight.

4. Water loss needs to be replaced.

5. Foods provide about one liter of fluid and the remainder must be obtained from drinks.

6. Water is needed for most body functions

Activity of water in the body:
1. It maintain the health and integrity of every cell in the body

2. It keeps the bloodstream liquid enough to flow through blood vessels.

3. It helps eliminate the by-products of the body's metabolism, excess electrolytes, for example sodium

and potassium, and urea, which is a waste product formed through the processing of dietary protein.

4. It regulates body temperature through sweating.

5. It keeps mucous membranes moist, such as those of the lungs and mouth.

6. It lubricates and cushions joints.

7. It reduces the risk of cystitis by keeping the bladder clear of bacteria.

8. It aids digestion and prevents constipation.

9. It works as a moisturizer to improve the skin's texture and appearance.

10. It carries nutrients and oxygen to cells.

11. It serves as a shock absorber inside the eyes, spinal cord and in the amniotic sac surrounding the fetus in pregnancy.

Water content in food
The article says that most foods, even those that look hard and dry, contain water. The body can get about half of its water needs from food alone. The digestion process also produces water as a by-product and can provide around 10 per cent of the body's water requirements. The rest must come from liquids ".

One final word, dehydration can result in nerve pain as the light fields in it find it difficult to move along the nerve pathway to where they are needed. Both the muscles and the nerves that pass through them as well as the organs they function through can produce a lot of pain from dehydration.

Chapter 3
Dehydration

The Better Health Channel BHC), a service fully funded by the State Government of Victoria (Australia) in their article on water [3-1] has the following to say about dehydration,

" Dehydration occurs when the water content of the body is too low. The good news is that this is a condition if identified can be easily fixed by increasing fluid intake.

Symptoms of dehydration include headaches, lethargy, mood changes and slow responses, dry nasal passages, dry or cracked lips, dark-colored urine, weakness, tiredness, confusion and hallucinations.

Eventually urination stops, the kidneys fail and the body can't remove toxic waste products. In extreme cases, this may result in death.

Causes of dehydration include (I have added information to give the computer use perspective to each cause identified by the BHC article):
1. Increased sweating due to hot weather, humidity, exercise or fever. This could also arise from the heat from computer screen light in some cases, as well as from the incandescent and fluorescent lights used to light up the room where the computer is being used.

2. Not drinking enough water. Many computer users are guilty of this. Many do not realize the constant feeling of thirst they feel while on the computer is a symptom of possible dehydration as a result of the light emanating from the computer screen.

To compound the problem many go for soda to quench their thirst instead of water.

3. Insufficient signaling mechanisms in the elderly –
    sometimes they do not feel thirsty even though they
    may be dehydrated. When elderly people are computer
    users, caregivers need to be aware that the issue of
    dehydration could be exacerbated

4. Increased output of urine due to a hormone deficiency,
    diabetes, kidney disease or medications.

    Any computer user who has any of these pre existing
    conditions will show more indication of these diseases
    because of the additional toxins they are exposed to in
    computer use and the dehydration arising from
    exposure to computer light.

    There will also be other issues due to neurotransmitter
    and nutrient depletions and so on inherent in computer
    use.

5. Diarrhea or vomiting.

6. Recovering from burns.

7. When you need to increase fluids

If a person regularly does not drink enough water there is
some increased risk of kidney stones and, in women,
urinary tract infections.

The article says that there is also limited evidence to
suggest an increased risk for some cancers including
bladder cancer and colon cancer. It can also lower a

person's physical and mental performance and salivary gland function.

Suffice to say that any pre existing condition will be exacerbated by computer use. This increase in symptoms can however be easily misdiagnosed and medicated with dire consequences as computer related issues do not resolve with medication.

They need to be addressed in a root cause treatment manner involving natural detoxification, nutrition, exercise, sun exposure and other targeted treatments that I have discussed in my various books.

The suggested solutions in this book addressed in chapter – 6- relate more specifically to the dehydration aspect of the problem.

To obtain information about solutions to other issues, please refer to books I have written on each issue. Also refer to my first 2 books – *Lessons I Learned the Hard Way* and *Computer Related Health Conditions.*

In addition, I have written 2 books on nutrition that address some of the nutritional issue – *Healing Juicing, Smoothie and Milk Shake Recipes* and *Healing Meals Recipes.*

The BHC article states that people who need more water in their diet include those who:

1. Are on a high protein diet

2. Are on a high fiber diet, as fluids help prevent constipation

3. Are children

4. Have an illness that causes vomiting or diarrhea

5. Are physically active

6. Are exposed to warm or hot conditions.

It is important that anyone with any of the identified risks for dehydration or who have kidney issues talk to their doctor about the effect of computer use on dehydration to avoid misdiagnosis, possible complications and over medication

Chapter 4
The computer use factor

Just as a hydroelectric power generation system needs water to conduct and generate electricity which it passes on to consumers, so our skin receptors, nasal passages, ears and eyes need to be hydrated for electrical fields to pass through them to our brains, hearts and other parts of our bodies where they are needed to empower us to carry out our daily functions as humans.

As we have read in this book, water is an essential component of our physical structure and a huge chunk of the composition of the brain is water.

Our brains are about 70 % water in weight. Need I say anything more about the importance of water? When dehydration occurs near the body's surrounding as occurs in computer use, it draws from our body through the skin and we feel dehydrated, uncomfortable

The composition of outdoor water that automatically continually rebalances itself is very different from that in enclosed environments, which is what we all live and work in today.

In addition, many of the materials used in building today's houses are cheap, artificially derived materials that are not in perfect synch with the natural outdoor environment.

This affects the quality of indoor air in every way including the moisture content.

The way buildings are built consequently means many of us spend most of the hours of everyday in enclosures that do not allow outdoor air in.

For example, in winter months in countries that experience cold seasons, the heater is on and many do not crack open their windows resulting in highly imbalanced and poor quality indoor air (a vaporizer is not a substitute for outdoor naturally moistened air. In my case using a vaporizer results in lung congestion).

The heater because of the heat makes it worse by drying up the already polluted and low quality air.

This is what results in a wide range of issues such as headaches, allergy and asthma like symptoms, dry eyes and other air quality related issues for computer users.

Such is the importance of good air moisture balance in the computer use environment.

Indeed the electrical currents that pass through the brain and that produce the energy for its function need water to pass through much like hydro electric power is generated.

The various light fields of word that power our bodies and that make up the body's messaging system we call neurotransmitters – a class of biochemicals, are passed from one part of the body to the other through the nerve network that must be well hydrated to function properly

Consequently, the issue of dehydration as a result of computer use is an important factor that affects our brain and nerve functions and consequently various aspects of our health.

It could also affect kidney function as the kidneys work to combat the toxins we are inherently exposed to in computer use.

In fact the very light emitting from the computer screen is toxic and contains many toxic chemicals and minerals that are in addition mainly artificially derived.

They are not normally found in nature in the form they are available in the computer screen and other computer parts we as humans are exposed to from computer use.

A good example of this is silicon, which only occurs in nature as silicon dioxide and which in addition only occurs in humans and animals in trace form and consequently is toxic to us in large quantities.

Computer use exposes us to silicon not as silicon dioxide but as pure silicon, which is contrary to the coded way we are supposed to be exposed to it. It is also in significant amount and not trace form as found in our bodies.

Computer use because of the toxins it exposes us to also probably makes the kidneys use up a lot of water in carrying out its detoxification process in the body during computer use.

The amount of fluid needed increases with the level of toxins. For example various websites have various colors and light field composition and an observant user will feel the effect in terms of things like varying rapid heart beats levels, excitement, level of concentration and so on.

In addition to this, light dries up moisture, which is why we feel thirsty in sunlight.

Though the heart and consequently the brain does not recognize the computer light as light evidenced by the fact that the blink function and other protective functions that are automatically switched on by the body when outside in sunlight fail to operate, the moisture drying activity still goes on as the light must pass through, be carried by and through moisture in the air for our eye nerves to receive it.

Light moves through moisture for it to be communicated to us.

Light is stressful to the body, however stress reducing auto functions including blinking that are automatically switched on in sunlight enable us handle the stress such that we actually calm down when in sunlight. Its rays empower our hearts to use our brain to produce inhibitory neurotransmitter that enable us to handle stress.

According to Dr. Larry K. Wan [4-1] we blink 66% less when in front of the computer. The malfunctioning of this stress reducing function that is critical to the body's ability to handle the stress of continual exposure to light is one of the many factors that result in the various stress related health issues experienced by computer users.

I will provide more details in the next chapter of the effect of dehydration from computer use on this body organ function.

Under normal conditions, our hearts stimulate our brains to produce inhibitory neurotransmitters such as Gamma Amino butyric Acid (GABA) to keep us calm in the presence of light. For light normally energizes us initiating the production of excitatory neurotransmitters of movement.

Unchecked and uncontrolled, we would over produce these excitatory neurotransmitters getting overly exited, in continual constant motion, feeling energized without restraint until we use up all the excitatory neurotransmitters and become unable for example to recognize danger or when we need to stop an action because we have for example used up all the adrenaline and noradrenaline in the system.

It is easy to get addicted to this overproduction of excitement and seek it continuously, which is how people get addicted to the computer.

It is indeed a sign of the depletion of the biochemicals that we call inhibitory neurotransmitters such as GABA that exercise control on our production of excitatory ones so we can function.

There are many mental and organ health issues associated with this depletion problem, making computer use a factor in the mental health of all computer users.

Depletion of inhibitory neurotransmitters is inherent in computer use but many do not recognize or even know about it.

All they know is that they feel empowered and excited on the computer and when away from it they feel empty. They also know that they feel compelled to sit in from of the computer and browse even if they have no need to be at the computer.

We also cut corners, drinking soda instead of water even when we know we should not do so and many of us are generally careless with our self control and our health unable to help ourselves because of the lack of resources needed to carry out the correct action.

That is why shouting and screaming at offenders to get off the computer and take a break many times may not work. They may be too depleted to carry out the necessary action to free themselves even though they may want to.

Indeed, the balance of neurotransmitters present in us at anytime determines our actions.

This happens with regular computers as well as computer gadgets like video games, cell phones (texting and sexting), ipads and so on.

We are unable to produce the inhibitors we need because only life containing light can stimulate us This we get from natural sources – the sun, moon an stars only. Computer light is not from a naturally luminous source and so is not life containing but lifeless and toxic.

Women, generally seem to get dehydrated very easily and carry bottles of water around. As a woman, I would suggest that it seems we feel dehydration faster than men or maybe they are not as aware of their bodies and when it hurts as we are.

Just as the light of the sun dehydrates us and we feel thirsty when walking on a sunny day so it is when we are in front of the computer.

Our skin and various receptors in them and the air around us become dehydrated. More so as most of us work in offices without windows or if they have windows they are kept permanently shut.

One area I have found that becomes very heavily affected is the skin at the sides of the eyes where the tear ducts are resulting in dry eyes from the drying of the muscles and the glands responsible for watering our eyes with tears i.e. the tear ducts.

The problem is exacerbated by the loss of blink function that would automatically normally water our eyes.

The moisturizers we women apply on our skin before makeup is good but not enough in addition, they contain several chemicals that may react with the chemicals in the computer monitor light to dehydrate our skin.

Lying on one's back periodically during the day with wet cotton balls placed on the eyelid and washing the face at least twice a day helps in keeping the skin around the eyes hydrated resulting in less dry eyes.

There is however a more effective way in the spraying of PH balanced water from which several chemicals and minerals have been removed.

The skin is able to absorb that more easily and it is much more effective in reducing dry eyes. For people who work in offices, this is a big help as it is unlikely one will be able to find anywhere in the office to lie down and do the wet cotton balls option.

I discovered this PH balanced water alternative when the manufacturers Bio-Logic Aqua Technologies International Inc. sent me some bottles of this water called Nature's Mist as a complementary gift for being on their radio show.

It was marketed as a product to help keep makeup in place all day by moisturizing the skin. I decided to give it a try instead as an aid for reducing dry eyes and found that it worked just fine. It is available on their website http://www.biologicaqua.com/home.php.

A second thing to do is to crack open the window and let the fresh air in. These two things complement each other and both need to be in place for maximum benefit. This may be something to discuss with your boss at the next meeting.

We will read more about this PH balanced water later in this chapter

Computer use induced dehydration and organ function
A large percentage of the human body weight as we have read, is water. In fact science as we have read many times in this book tells us that our brains are 70% water. The electrical currents that operate our body systems need water for transmission. That is how we understood how to generate hydroelectric power supply.

If our bodies get dehydrated the normal electrical transmission system in our bodies could be affected and we begin to feel uncomfortable as the biochemical supply in various body parts are depleted as the receptors malfunction from the lack of hydration.

When we sit before a computer, the light and electrical charges that emit from the screen enable us to see the objects on the screen, they also dehydrate the surrounding area consequently dehydrating our skins when we sit in offices where there is no natural ventilation

Natural outside air is coded to continuously rehydrate itself. This natural process is lost in closed window environments resulting in a feeling of discomfort when we work for long periods in such environment due to the effect of the dehydration on the electrical transmission systems in our bodies starting from our skin and into the inward part of our systems.

More on the effect on the eyes and brain functions
As we have read, the dehydration of the skin around our eyes I have discovered is the reason for the dry eyes symptoms we sometimes feel during and after computer use.

That is why eye drops do not help. Washing the face regularly helps but I have discovered that spraying specially PH balanced water we read about earlier on the facial skin gives a much more dramatic and longer lasting effect. This is because atmospheric water has a different PH from that of tap water.

I discovered that after a few days of use my chronic dry eyes that had resisted all other solutions became almost non-existent.

I hope we can see the importance of water to the computer user. We need to drink water to meet the frequent thirsty feelings (not soda) and ensure adequate skin hydration.

It is important to note that without access to outside fresh air that can easily be achieved by cracking open the windows, we will not achieve enough hydration to achieve optimal body and brain function and consequently work productivity.

It is important to locate our home computers close to the window to allow fresh air to come in.

Anyone who has been in an arid environment knows the discomfort that comes from being in a low moisture content environment.

It affects the thinking capability and other decision making processes.

It brings on irritability and an inability to cope with normal day to day functions that are easier to handle in a well moistened environment.

The body is able to easily recalibrate itself when water is provided when dehydration does not have the added issue of toxic light and other imbalances in the environment due to operating computers or computer devices.

In that case the restoration is slower and takes consistent effort over time including an effort to avoid other stresses and toxins to allow the boy to build up its resources.

Chapter 5
The Resulting Health Issues

Body organs
As we have read in this book, computer use puts more pressure on our kidneys and livers to remove toxins from our bodies.

That is why after using the computer for about an hour the urine becomes darker from both dehydration and the concentration of toxins being eliminated.

This could result in higher creatinine and metal levels in the urine and blood as the kidney becomes over burdened and unable to fully carry out its normal function effectively.

Someone who discovered their urine becoming cloudy consulted me a few years ago for help. Others have spoken of being diagnosed with mild kidney problems.

To compound matters, a factor many do not realize is that there are some minerals that are heavily used up during computer use notably iron which is heavily used by the body anytime it is in the presence of light. Magnesium, calcium, vitamin B, D and other nutrients involved in the reading and information processing functions are also implicated.

Consequently, the effect of dehydration from computer use is complicated by mineral and biochemical depletions that could easily result in a misdiagnosis of the reason for many ailments that afflict computer users.

Computer use makes us multitask on a continual basis for long periods of time contrary to the way our body carries out our normal human living body function

Iron, a mineral heavily used up in the computer use activity for example is a key part of the composition of the blood. In addition it helps to maintain our body temperature and prevents us from being fried up by the sunlight.

It is also just below the surface of the earth's crust in high concentrations regulating the temperature of the earth's crust and involved in the gravity function hat helps to keep us on the earth and able to walk on it. It prevents the earth's crust from over heating.

It is part of the component of the body's moisture that helps in absorbing sunlight hence the more pigmented we are, the more we can absorb sunlight and the inhibitors we need from the sun that help to keep us alive.

When the body is dehydrated, all these function fail to operate properly for water is the medium through which all these activities take place.

The code of nature
As we have read in this book, Nature's user manual tells us the earth was initially covered with water. When time came for the earth to be revealed external light was provided, its water was split into two.

This split created a system of a cover of water above the earth cooling the earth, while mist was on the actual surface of the land and there were seas and rivers.

This system was very conducive and the iron from the plant source that was the initial food of humans was enough to sustain life here on earth.

After the first rain with the flood of Noah's days, the system of hydrating the earth was change to that of clouds, rain, seas, rivers and oceans.

The loss of the cooling system of the water above that was replaced with clouds, which are much lighter resulted in the iron source being insufficient to handle the effect of direct exposure to sunlight and the need for more inhibitory neurotransmitters to handle the stress.

Because these changes were brought about by our maker flexibilities were automatically brought into play to handle the situation,

Human were allowed to eat meat to obtain additional amino acids, iron and enzymes needed for survival in the new environment.

The change, which would have been devastating, was not.

This is the only way to have changes to the system that flow in line with the rest of nature. Our maker must orchestrate it directly and put in the flexibilities and changes required.

Consequently, computer use is something we have put in place without asking for help. It is a user defined configuration change allowed to the system that requires either the programmer to fix the code to handle the changes or help us identify things he has already put in nature to enable us handle this change without a direct fix to the code.

This is the missing link in today's innovation and why instead of solving problems we do not solve anything with our innovation but create new problems.

Everything we do is like introducing software not configured into a system into it or introducing a computer virus with the potential to destroy the system.

It is in fact the misuse of the privilege of choice.

Our maker already anticipated we would carry out all we are doing today and in his mercy has put in nature systems to ensure this dangerous tool would not result in our self destruction when we unleash it.

Consequently when we do our part of acknowledging him and his authority and humble ourselves to ask him to show is what he has put in nature for such a time as this, he shows us we do it and everything flows in synch.

Some of what I learned by doing this, which is how I was able to recover from life threatening health issues arising from my many years of incessant computer use is what I share in this book and all my other books.

I have done this in order to help others to receive the healing I received and continue to enjoy so they too can have their situations turned around no matter how bad things have become like mine was.

My computer use is now a long term blessing and not a long term curse as it became several years ago (refer to my book – *Lessons I Learned the Hard Way*)

We will now go back to the subject at hand. When there was a cover of water, there was no need for the specific activities of the sun and moon we have today that results in formation of clouds.

There was only a need for activities that resulted in a mist that watered the ground that in turn resulted in the growth of plants. Everything was easy.

Indeed the need for the continual water cover is why we have clouds and rain, which all depend on the wind and the activities of the sun and moon.

And as we have read in this book, anything made from the earth needs water to survive. It needs it for emitting light so it can be seen and also for taking in light.

That is one of the reasons why dry scalps, hair and skin are so problematic

The Eyes and Skin
Without water the body loses it ability to receive neurotransmitters via the light receptors that become unable to function properly and this could in turn result in an inability to properly emit light leading to fatality if water is not quickly provided to the dehydrated person.

It could also lead to infection of the receptors and nerves. I suffered severe infection no one could diagnose or treat.

In computer use, this need for hydration as we have read, is the reason why the drying of the skin around the eyes as a result of computer light, results in dry eyes.

Outside air has a very different PH from that in tap water consequently, washing the face and applying moisturizers alone does not resolve this dry eyes phenomenon neither does applying eye drops.

The only thing I have found from experience that works as at the time of writing (December 2012/January 2013) as I have written in this book and my other books is Nature's Mist from Bio-Logic Aqua Technologies International Inc – Special Natural Spring water that has a certain PH.

I at the time I discovered it was what I needed for my dry eyes was shopping around for water with a PH close to that of outside air. Our maker from the manual had shown me my dry eyes issues were the effect of computer light on the skin around my eyes and that the only solution was to have the water levels of the skin restored.

As I said earlier on in this book, I decided to see if it was what I was looking for. It worked perfectly and I have used it since.

My dry eyes that had been so bad I had not shed tears for months totally vanished within a few weeks of intensive use. I urge you to try it.

Daily use by spraying it on the face before washing, the face and spraying it on as needed while using the computer, will gradually completely heal your dry eye syndrome. I have recommended it to many people with the same result every time. It works.

There is also something to remember when it comes to the ability of the skin to absorb sunlight which is critical for maintaining human life and which supplies us with the ability to produce inhibitory neurotransmitters that enable us to operate as humans.

Less pigmented people are unable to take in as much light i.e. inhibitors as pigmented people, leading to their having more difficulty in being calm.

Statistics (for more details please get hold of my book "computer use induced stress") indicate that the rate of depression is higher in less pigmented people. Hence though every computer user needs to ensure they get adequate daily sunlight, less pigmented people must make double sure.

You do not need to stand in the sun directly for too long as you do not have the protection of pigmentation, which is the natural protection that prevents the rays from destroying the skin while being absorbed.

It also ensures that the light that comes in stays in and is not lost i.e. it aid retention.

To protect itself skin with less pigmentation is unable to absorb and retain the light fields in the amounts needed without malfunctioning (called melanoma or skin cancer over time).

If you are out in the sun for long you may need something with Sun Protection Factor (SPF).

The eyes also need daily exposure to sunlight but after some time people with blue or grey or other low pigmented iris may need to wear sunglasses for part of the time.

Do what is appropriate for your pigmentation level.

Inadequate sunlight exposure could result in computer use induced mental issues that will not get resolved without a sun exposure therapy in addition to other holistic measures.

Chapter 6
Suggested Practical Solutions

Here are some practical easy things that all computer users should also consider adopting as preventive measures to ensure adequate hydration and sunlight exposure in addition to all the measures already discussed

Dehydration Preventive Measures

1. Drink water often during computer use. Keep in tune with your body so you can detect when you are thirsty

    :

    The importance of water to optimal functioning of our body system cannot be overemphasized. In fact the electrical fields in us need the water to pass through just as when electricity is generated from hydroelectric sources.

    It is consequently important to drink water during computer use. Do not allow the pressure of deadline make you ignore the thirsty feelings that come. If you do, do not be surprised if you feel totally spent, irritable, and light headed, absent-minded and/or forgetful when you leave the computer.

2. Your digestive system may also take a hit. You must however combine your water intake with exercise to improve circulation. Excessive water intake could make you tired and feel weighed down. If this happens, do some exercise to encourage your body to eliminate the excess. Please note that soda and other drinks are not good substitutes for plain water.

3. Avoid Soda.

4. Use a hydrating moisturizer.

5. Use Nature's Mist by Bio Logic Aqua LLC to heal and to prevent dry eyes.

6. Wash your face at the end of the day after computer use to wash away the toxins that have clung to the skin.

7. Crack open your window to allow fresh air in to ensure continual rebalancing of air moisture as happens with outside air.

8. Make one day in the week a computer free day. Make this a weekly habit and you will notice an immediate effect the first week.

9. Have a computer free vacation.

10. Use an air purifier with ionizer. This only works when you crack open your windows as well. Purifiers need access to fresh air to be effective and the ones I have used actually have this fact stated in the instruction book that comes with them. Please refer to my book *"lessons I Learned the Hard Way"* for more on this issue.

11. Place green indoor plants in the room where your computer is so they can absorb the carbon dioxide co2 that your computer emits.

12. Go for daily walks. Drink water before and after your walk

13. Do indoors and outdoors stretching exercises. Also exercise your face. Drink water after exercising.

14. Do indoors and outdoors eye exercises letting your eyes see far out from all the corners of your eyes to exercise the eye muscles.

15. Read daily outside with the light of the sun letting the eyes operate in the natural way it was code to. You will find your eyes beginning to improve if you do this consistently no matter how old you are. I find reading the manual for the use of the systems of nature that we call the Bible gives the best result.

Here are other tips for general good computer use health

16. Eat organic to avoid additional toxic chemicals since you are exposed to enough of them through computer use. The less the toxins the body is exposed to the better it performs.

17. Eat plenty of fruits and vegetables.

18. Cook with Olive Oil (pure olive oil for cooking and extra virgin for salads and other things that you do not apply heat to) or use organic Canola oil.

19. Take organic grass fed milk and not regular milk. If you are unable to find this you may take organic almond milk or rice milk or goat milk

20. Eat only meat from organic grass fed cows and lamb. Goat is wild so that should be okay. Red meat has more easily digestible iron and plenty of the enzymes and amino acid that computer users need. This is why vegetarians may find themselves constantly weak.

The red meat is not the problem and is what we actually need with the high exposure to all this light in the technology age. Cow and other animals were however only coded to eat grass and their bowels cannot fully digest grains and so the undigested grain in their system is what gives the gas and other issues.

If you eat organic grass fed red meat you will find yourself healing fast. Humans are the problem not the animals. Try organic grass fed Bison and other game i.e. eat only meat not tampered with by humans. Remember to eat the organs and the skin (the skin is where the collagen is).

There is more to say on this but maybe in another book dedicated to meats for compute users

21. Eat organic eggs for easily absorbable iron and vitamin B Complex. Eating egg however requires that you take fluid for ease of digestion.

22. Also eat only wild caught fish (remember the skin has the most nutrient do not throw it away) and other sea food.

23. Consult with your doctor about possible need to supplement your iron, magnesium, and vitamin B, D, C and Calcium if you are suffering from the consequences of dehydration. Also consult with your doctor about taking a good multivitamin containing a good combination of micronutrients.

24. Doctors please refer to my book Lessons I Learned the Hard way for advice on supplementing amino acids to resolve depletion of GABA, Melatonin and so on.

Computer users, please do not self diagnose and supplement. Work with your doctor to avoid serious complications and possible interactions with drugs you are taking for other issues.

25. In addition avoid anything that is genetically modified. Eat only things in the state they were created to be. For example eat only seeded fruits. Fruits were made to have seeds.

   That is how the life is passed on. Hence seedless versions have some missing elements that may be critical for us as humans.

   The process of making them seedless has interfered with a natural process, which means the fruit is no longer in the way the human body is configured to receive and process it.

   Today everyone is saying it does not matter. Trust me, some years from now this will be identified as why for example certain cancers, diabetes and so on are in existence or killing people.

26. Your doctor should monitor you. Go for your regular check up.

27. Go for an annual eye exam to catch eye issues before they become a big problem.

28. Consider using ginger, garlic, onions and cayenne pepper in your food and adding them to your daily juice intake.

29. If you have constipation issues, blending your fruit into a juice by adding hot/boiling water may improve

absorption and assist the breakdown of fecal waste as well as partially pasteurize your juice in order to kill the bacteria and other germs from handling. It may be a good idea to try this. That is what I do

30. I will repeat, avoid genetically modified foods. The assurances people are being given today of their safety are destined to be turned into cancer scares down the road. Protect yourself.

Chapter 7
Summary

The user manual for the earth we call the Bible or Scriptures tell us that in the beginning, the earth was submerged in water and not visible as there was not enough light for that. All that was detectible in nature was the electromagnetic field of sound. This made the presence of water known. Everything else was hidden in darkness.

The earth did not have enough light in itself to be visible. It did not exist in the visible real but it was hidden in the water.

Consequently water is very critical to our very existence since we are made from the dust of the earth. Anything made from the earth therefore needs moisture around it to function. That is how the earth was preserved from its beginning and consequently inadequate water on the surface of the earth and anything made from it would be disastrous and affect its very existence.

Here is what the manual says in layman's English - There was darkness over the face of the land. Then the maker coded external light separate from the objects in existence, which had only the light in themselves able to make them exist.

This external light made it possible to see what had been hidden.

For example, the water in which the earth had been submerged was made visible. It was no longer just sound.

It also exposed darkness which had been the norm as being weak unable to keep its territory until the maker made some changes to ensure existence of darkness in order to create time and the solid bodies of the thing in nature.

For objects are formed from coding light to emit out of darkness in certain configurations of coding to form the various objects we see.

These various changes was all positive and had no destructive side effect as it was brought about by the maker who alone knows the programming language, can see it, has control over it, designed the code and knows the purpose for the whole of existence.

His changes flowed perfectly with the existing code of nature and was a perfect fit. It was not an attempt by one of the systems within the global system of nature that had been assigned limited control getting over its head into what it did not know.

From our activities as humans using the Hebrew mathematical symbols to write codes, we know that only the person who has the source code can make changes to the code of a system. Anyone else would only be creating chaos.

This is the simple reason why none of our advancement has resulted in the desired goal of solving any problems. We have never solved any and have only created new ones that never existed before we tampered with systems we knew nothing about.

We have gone beyond ourselves since we are not the writer of the code of nature but one of the many systems within the system of nature that is currently malfunctioning at a rapid pace towards self destruction.

Indeed, the only part we have access to with our codes is the lifeless physical/physiological part, which is the end result and not the unseen part that controls everything.

We are therefore making changes at the end product level, which may not be compatible with the level where the actual controls that govern things actually exist and operate from. Consequently we only unleash havoc at the end product level.

The Hebrew writings were only given to my ancestors to enable them understand nature and our maker, understand and appreciate his love and not for attempting to tamper with things to see how we can circumvent the controls put in place for our good.

What we have done is gone ahead without permission in rebellion to attempt to get away from the very controls that ensure we exist. We have been allowed to do our worst much like we allow rebellious kids to do their worst because that is the only way they will learn.

We do not really do anything constructive though we may fool other human and ourselves for a time until what we have done begins to unravel or creates serious havoc we are unable to resolve.

We as humans have been careless with our health and under the wrong assumption that we can do whatever we want without paying a price for it.

Apparently that is not so. It would seem that whatever we do must be within the code of nature for it to be seamless.

When we violate the code of nature we end up hurting ourselves and find that sometimes we cannot turn back what we have unleashed and are stuck with the problems we have created in the quest of solving some other problem.

It seems our search for solutions using technology has only considered the monetary gains and ability to use the perceived knowledge to exercise dominion over others.

Little consideration if any is given to the downside of the cost to nature and the violations in our technology of our natural coded way of being with its consequent toll on human health and other parts of nature.

In many cases we have become penny wise and pound foolish.

There seems to be a lack of depth of knowledge about codes and how they work despite being a generation of humans that have most of our innovation based on codes.

We talk about genetic codes, DNA codes and so on without thinking of the significance of what we are saying.

What it means is an environment or product based on specific terms and conditions and that can only operate as intended based upon those terms and conditions being maintained 100 percent.

Any changes will make the product or environment to malfunction and self destroy.

For it to adjust to any change the flexibility must have been written into the script by the programmer or else the system will malfunction.

Only the programmer can make successful changes into the system or product.

Since we humans are coded beings, it means we are the product of written scripts that have a beginning and an end i.e. that has a definite specific outcome.

We have flexibility provided in our scripts. We cannot amend our codes. It can only be amended by our programmer/developer.

We may talk about DNA or genetic code to impress other humans but it means nothing but a guesswork game for we profess to know so much about what we know nothing and can never know anything about as what we profess to know can only be known by our maker who has scripted boundaries in us to ensure we remain in existence.

Any code must have its beginning and end and every stage that is in between in place before it can function.

In addition, only our programmer who designed us can make changes in our code. Anything we claim to be doing is really operating as malfunctioning machines and not making any change to any code.

That is why all our experiments are all hurting us and destroying us and the environment we live in, because changes have to be done by our maker or under his direction before they can work.

He must put in the flexibility first before things can be okay.

Our self delusionary theory of evolution has made us believe our lies can change things.

The truth is that the theory of evolution is not compatible with the operation of codes for codes must be spoken and written by someone. They are defined and controlled environments that operate on absolute truth.

A code will only do what the code says regardless of the intent. The code is in absolute control over what it produces. There cannot be random codes. Codes are specific. They do not evolve.

Codes cannot evolve but must follow a predetermined set of rules. Codes must be controlled. It is the controls that ensure that the predetermine end is achieved. Without the controls in place that ensure that anything not within the code or given flexibility by the code will fail, it would not achieve the desired purpose.

That is why for example plastic does not biodegrade. Its component is not recognized by the code of the biodegrade process that determines how things are biodegraded in nature.

When we make artificial things that are not made under the directive of the master, which consequently he has not provide flexibility for, or maybe he has provided for it in the manual but humans are trying to achieve that end outside of the constraint of the controls put in place, then it will not work.

This is all why the computer use environment hurts. We have decided to go beyond the intended use of the system without the input of the maker in foolish greed to our own detriment.

Consequently, though the system is useful and helps us understand our creator more, any expansion of its use beyond just a better knowledge of our maker into actual daily functionality needs the direct okay and input by our maker to make it compatible with the existing system in an operational mode.

We should have acknowledged and consulted with he who alone knows the end result of creation and how to arrive there.

Because we failed to do this, we have in place a system that violates our natural coded way of being.

It is obvious certain preventive measures must be put in place or certain changes made to the existing code of our being to prevent the violations inherent in our innovations from hurting us.

The manual tells us we are made from word that it is a written code that operates in us to make us who we are.

Science agrees with it. For cells do not communicate directly with each other and have no life of their own but are controlled by word we call a class of biochemicals called neurotransmitters that are constantly relaying messages from cell to cell and all around the body. They are responsible for passing life to the cells

This is much like the electricity from the switch being passed though certain magnetic fields that operates the commands of the Hebrew mathematical symbols that we write as codes to manifest what we see on the computer screen.

The word of the code is how the system receives the light currents and fields that result in what we see on the screen.

These symbols my ancestors told the world was provided by the God of the Bible who wrote the code of our being. These symbols however only work on things within the jurisdiction that we are given.

There are other spoken words used by today's descendants of the Jews of old in all of sub-Saharan Africa, which was the science of these people before they convinced themselves the European way was easier and consequently lost a lot of that science which would have immensely helped us today if we still had the knowledge.

Chapter 8
Making Technological advancement non destructive

I am going to do something in this book, I have never done in any of my other books on computer use induced health conditions – get to the root of why our technology is so destructive. Why we are never able to achieve our aim of a better system of nature and human structure.

Each new advancement is more destructive than the prior one. Something is missing and very badly wrong fundamentally.

If you are beginning to feel uneasy, I advice you to ignore the feeling and read on. That feeling is a sign that you know you are about to be hit with the truth and you will have to decide whether to live or continue on the path of destruction.

It is also a sign that the thought you are having is originating from darkness and the source of it is afraid of being exposed by the light of the truth. This is your chance for self-deliverance. Take it and be free. Read on.

The code of nature like every other code is precise and controlled. It is the controls put in a code by the programmer that ensures that the desired end result is achieved.

Hence the controls in nature that prevent us from having our way are what ensure that we do not destroy ourselves or any other thing entirely from our often foolish actions providing a means for the system to self correct.

The manual tells us that the end result in the case of the production code for the product called the earth and all that is within it, is to go from an earth unseen and covered by water and darkness to one that is filled with light and life such that it shines brighter than the sun in its brightness and is everlasting and eternal.

It has currently been placed in and is indeed going through a process of refinement orchestrated by our maker to achieve this end, which is why we have had and still have so many issues on earth as the manual tells us will happen.

Refinement is a hard process that removes all dross or impurity or baggage to reveal the gem or pure metal that is precious and pure.

Let us try and understand just one of the systems in nature, the human body.

Each cell in our body is a complex system. It is like having a computer system that has in it over 100 million kinds of software operating simultaneously on several millions of hardware all connected together whose electrical current is generated through and passed through a continuous flow of water.

If we have about 4 billion cells as science tells us imagine how complex the human body is. That is why no one can repair it. It must self-repair as our maker has designed it. Anything we put in must flow in line with the coded self repair system kit to work.

That is what the medical profession is about. It is about trying to firstly correctly identify the repair kit for various ailments and secondly identify the various components so when we supply them, the body is empowered to repair itself.

This is why medications we engineer outside of natural processes have all the various side effects and very often fail to work over time as the self repair kit's resources becomes overwhelmed trying to fit the bad software we have engineered into the process.

This is also why being dehydrated is not an option.

The human system is just one of the myriads of systems in nature. There are systems we can see naturally and those we cannot see which are more powerful than those we can see and which control what we see.

Water for example is not all physical. There is an unseen part of it. Neither is dehydration only physical. There is also an unseen part of every ailment and of everything else.

Read along to fully understand this concept.

The system of nature as we can see is super complex, more than any human brain can fathom or try to comprehend.

That is why our maker is the only command because such a complex system cannot be left to others except the programmer who put it all together to achieve his purpose.

Each system has a part to play in the grand design.

Consequently, only our maker is able to control, controls things and orchestrates things in nature in accordance with the code of nature, which he put in place before bringing everything forth.

This is what we try to copy with technology. We first decide what we want to produce and why i.e. the purpose it will achieve. Then we design the code, anticipate all the processes required to achieve the desired end product as well as all the scenarios that can go wrong and provide processes for correcting them in such a way that the end result is still accomplished.

Indeed as we have read in this book, before a code can be successfully run it must have an end and a beginning and all the possible situations and steps needed to go from beginning to the end must be anticipated before hand and coded in.

Anything that comes up later that was not anticipated must be put in by the programmer for the code to successfully go beyond the point where the anomaly was introduced.

The fact that the code of nature goes on regardless of what the various systems do and it self corrects and self eliminates all bottle necks tells us all things happening were anticipated before the code started running and everything is going on as planned to arrive at the coded end.

This is good news for us because it means there is a solution for every problem we can possibly have as individuals, corporations, as families, nations or even globally. The code will run its course. We will either be on the side that is preserved in the course of correction or eliminated.

The beauty of it all is that we have a good maker who does not want anything to be destroyed and will show us the way out if we acknowledge him. He will not stop the code for he has set a date certain for the end product to manifest. He will however ensure we do not self destroy unless we choose to.

That is why everyone has a choice. Each choice however has a consequence and the code for the consequence of each action will run when we make them so we must be careful to weigh the consequence before acting.

Some actions have rewind functions and some do not.

Everything is connected together by one thing that is common to all - life.

Life is what our maker uses to control and connect all things consequently anything that does not have life will not flow in synch with nature.

This life is coded to flow through from point to point through a seamless combination of seen and unseen water systems. Life is light. It is the light of life that controls all things.

This is why all our lifeless innovation is problematic to the natural environment and ourselves

Non destructive innovation
The only way to make technological advancement non-destructive is to invite the maker to lead the way and get involved.

He alone can make changes to the code of nature or else show us what preventive measures we need to put in place that he has already provided in nature to enable us avoid being destroyed by what we are doing.

He alone controls life and without life being introduced into what we do it will never flow in synch with nature but will be a virus and a destructive force in nature as all our innovations today are.

We cannot operate without life and everything it needs to operate such as water. We have no access to light or life for they do not originate in the physical but the spiritual realm our maker alone has access to.

The artificial light we produce is not from nothing it is from something already existing but not coded to be self-luminous. Hence its light has no life.

Unless we can produce our own nature from scratch that will exist without life and water or anything else we cannot come up with, and unless we can recreate ourselves from scratch from nothing, we will never be able to do anything non destructive without the maker's input.

Accepting that in humility is the beginning of the solution.

Life as it is light also needs both seen and unseen water to pass through. That is the code, which we cannot change or affect.

Let us now get an understanding of how we got into this mess.

We humans like to think we have knowledge but actually no one has thoughts of their own but receive thoughts.

Hence when we accept anyone's ideas we are actually accepting the ideas of the source of their thoughts either light or darkness.

Consequently, what passes for knowledge and which may seem logical may be deception. It may actually work for some time but sooner than later it will begin to fail.

That is why our science is always changing because it is coming from deceptive sources. One person gets deceived and he or she convinces the rest to accept the deceptive thoughts they have received.

Some of this so called knowledge and "deceptive" science is a deliberate attempt to deceive in order to maintain an economic advantage. Some of it is a result of ego and pride, taking advantage of others because they show themselves gullible even when it is obvious what is being proposed is a lie.

The temptation to deceive increases when the recipients proceed to swallow everything they are told without questioning the source of the lies. It emboldens the deceiver

We all know that life is not physiological and cannot be seen or tested though it may seem like a nice thought to be able to see life and be in control of it. This leaves us open to deception and to be willing to accept deceptive thoughts received by others as fact.

Anyone who is always looking for knowledge out of curiosity will always be open to deception. The only way to avoid deception is to know the truth and to always weigh everything against the truth. The first thing to do is understand that people have no thought of their own. The first course of action is to check the source of their thoughts.

Are they in any occult group or fraternities? How do they receive their thoughts? Where do the thoughts they receive come from?

For example we have a chemical we call **Deoxyribonucleic acid** (DNA). This is an acid i.e. a chemical with acidic property and which can be extracted. Acids react with other chemicals. These are all physical things. Life is not physical. It does not react with chemicals to produce anything. It is not carbon.

When people say DNA has the genetic code for life. Can that be possible or is not that just wishful thinking.

It is possible to have a chemical that reacts in peculiar way with certain fluids in a specific way, which may be a way of identifying a person or their relatives. It does not mean that is the code of life.

All it means is that certain fluids are passed from generation to generation. We pass everything we are over to others. The balance of coded word in each person is passed down.

It also means some reaction with chemicals of saliva and other fluids from the body can also give an indication when compared with those of others who have the same disease and so on what diseases and so on they have inherited.

That is very different from the code of a person's life. It is only an indication that certain people are related.

It does not show the code of their lives. That is something that is not physiological and not a chemical.

The code of life will show what a particular person was designed to be. No chemical can show that.

The language we humans speak cannot be seen. We can hear but cannot see the words we speak for these are light field. Though we cannot see these words we can see their affect in the physical realm, which is the realm we operate in and can see as humans.

We are all aware that the realm of the words we speak is different from the realm of their effect, which is what we see. The realm we cannot see consequently controls that we do see.

The coded word of our makeup is written in the unseen realm in a language we cannot see or hear and the effect of it such as human flesh and human actions is what we see

Coded words do not react with chemicals. Words are light fields. Only coded word in the physical realm we are given some control over can be written and seen as written words by us.

However the coded realm that controls us is out of our range. The only glimpse of it is we have is the manual of our being we call the Bible or Scriptures which is the interpretation of the unseen code of our being translated into human language we can hear and understand and write into letters we can read.

It is given to us to empower us with the truth so we do not fall into deception but avoid and challenge it when it shows up. Hence a guide for avoiding deception is to check every thought or so called knowledge people tell us with it.

Even neurotransmitters the words that operate us and other biochemicals cannot be seen.

We only see their effect because they are word. No one has ever seen any word. We only see the effect of a word that we write as code. The Hebrew mathematical symbols given to my ancestors by our maker, which he empowered to instruct light fields to carry out certain commands cannot be seen in real sense we only see something written to represent them but no one has ever seen any electromagnetic field or light.

We can use chemicals to stain a surface to give us the possible paths of their activities but it may not be the real thing even if some assumptions we make based on what we see seem to be working.

The fact that many of our assumptions we seem so sure about fail later tells us we were not seeing what we thought we were seeing in the first place for we cannot see the light fields themselves.

The true science are the scientific Hebrew writings which are the enlightenment our maker gave to my ancestors thousands of years ago based on their study of the manual we call the Bible or Scriptures (in those days they were called the law and the prophets).

Today's scientific innovations that work are from these writings. No one is doing anything new.

In fact the story is told that when Sir Isaac Newton who introduced us to modern physics died and people visited his apartment hoping to find out the secret of his knowledge, they did not find experiments. All they found were copies of the Hebrew writings and the manual we call the Bible or Scriptures.

All he did was compare the writings to the manual and then made them available as new scientific findings. That was what Science was for thousands of years just confirming the Hebrew writing.

In today's world in a bid for economic advantage, we have gone a step further, actually implementing the ideas without a go ahead from the maker, in defiance believing it is okay for whatever we come up with to operate only in the physical, that somehow the controlling realms will yield to us without the maker's input.

As we read in earlier chapters our assumptions were not right. The maker is in the driver's seat and not us.

When we say we do genetic engineering. It is just playing with chemicals to see its effect. We do not do anything to any code.

This grand deception and the willingness of people to be deceived into thinking humans are more than they are has made fortunes for people at the expense of the lives of others.

This is because people want to be powerful and in control and superior i.e. humans want to be their own God and maker, which is why we are all in the current problem of computer use induced health conditions.

When we receive a few thoughts that answer our curiosity about something we claim it to be ours instead of giving credit to our maker who has provided the information.

In private we marvel at how great God is but then in public and in our papers and writings we do not give him the glory and we allow other humans to heap praise on us which then opens us to the temptation of going beyond what we have received to receiving deception so we can continue to make more and more money.

With this knowledge of the foundation of our problem let us look at the manual for guidance.

What we need to remember from our user manual
In the beginning, the earth was without form and void. It was not. It was coded from reversing the code of light to form darkness and making this darkness to emit light in a way to form solid objects that could be visible with the provision of high density external light Nobody knew what the earth was like or would be until our maker pulled back the water to reveal it

It is this principle that guided our ability to develop an earth like environment in The **National Aeronautics and Space Administration** (NASA) space station that human astronauts live in.

As long as they stay inside it they can exist in space. When they go outside to repair the station they have to wear suits that have earth like oxygen laden environment to survive. If they for one moment peep out of it they would automatically be destroyed.

That is because anything in anyway different from the atmosphere on earth is toxic and indeed lethal for humans. We cannot survive above the highest mountain peak for land is require for the presence of oxygen in the amounts required for land oriented beings.

Fish is specially equipped to be able to source its oxygen from water. Birds are specifically equipped to be able to generate oxygen at levels where there is little or none in a special coded way provided for them by the maker.

Each species is designed for its environment in a way to protect them from other species.

The bird runs away from danger by flying away, fish by swimming away, animals on land by running faster than the adversary.

Everything is designed to respect and fear humans and humans are designed to take care of everything here.

As long as each remains where they are supposed to be there is no problem but when territories are invaded, confusion sets in as we have on earth today. Humans brought about the confusion and we are responsible for restoring things or else we will go extinct with everything else we are disturbing.

Just as the ability to kill others is not a license to kill but an opportunity to develop good character, the ability to go to space and other things we do is not a license for us to do so and cause confusion and self destruction but an opportunity to develop self control, understand our maker and choose to self preserve and stay humble and not take liberty for license to oppress and destroy as we are doing.

A huge portion of our climate change problem arises from our space travel for all the petroleum products and other things we introduce there are toxic to that environment which controls ours so when we poison the source of our environment, our environment becomes poisoned.

The question of carbon emission and so on we are trying to tackle is only a small part of the problem.

Gravity was given to us to enable us exercise restraint upon our knowledge. Our maker lets us choose but there are consequences for everything we do as the manual tells us and we are supposed to weigh the consequence of self annihilation against the satisfaction of the curiosity to find out whether we will self destroy or not.

A cessation of space venture will soon be forced upon us by the system in self preservation unless we heed the warnings of global warning which is a way of the systems in the heavenlies telling us to stay away or else---

The Long term Global Solution
A major issue we have is that our science is derived from the Hebrew writing that our maker gave to my ancestors the real Jews (black people with kinky hair).

Only they can really receive from the maker because that is how he has coded it. The manual tells us that my people are the light and salt of the earth and that salvation will only be brought into the earth through them.

Unfortunately, everybody else has decided they can also carry out this function that is not coded in them to achieve.

Consequently the end product of their venturing into bringing the various things in the Hebrew writings forth is corrupted and does not achieve the end of truly being a benefit.

There is no shortcut. The real Jews must be encouraged to take back their identity and fulfill their role that no one else can fulfill. You need the pigmentation to be able to receive the light and the wooly hair to be identified as the maker's sheep to whom alone belongs the knowledge by covenant.

The manual tells us others will try and fulfill the role of my people but will fail.

We the people on the earth at this time all have a choice, we either fall in line with the manual and receive the salvation we are all looking for, or continue on the current path to self destruction.

The many shootings we have today resulting from mental impairment is one of the many examples of the problem.

There is something common with all the shooters. They are all avid computer users. If some of us did not know dehydration and toxicity have negative consequences for brain function we all now know this from reading this book and thereby getting to understand the link between computer use, toxicity, dehydration and brain function.

There is a solution and our maker is able to make it known. The fact that I have been able to receive all the information in my various books is evidence of the fact that our maker is still willing to save all through my people the real Jews.

However for so long my people have been prevented from acknowledging themselves and the whole earth has suffered the consequence. As I have said the pigmentation and the kinky hair is for a purpose and it cannot be replaced as that is the code.

The current way of trying to use them without acknowledging who they are will not work. They can only be light if they operate as who they are, content to be different from others not trying to be like others and go directly through the manual themselves without interference from others.

They must be willing to do the hard work of getting to know the maker directly and being his sheep as they were coded to be. The kinky hair is the sheep hair that identifies them in the heavenlies.

The pigmentation enables them to absorb enough physiological light so they have enough light fields to receive the light of the words from the maker directly without being destroyed by it and without it being corrupted.

That is why they are the only ones he could make a covenant with. They alone have the physiological requirement for the spiritual light to operate through.

We humans are three dimensional. We are each made up of - The Spirit, which is unseen, connects us to our maker, is a part of him and is light and life where there is no darkness or death at all, The physical flesh that is visible darkness that has no light and consequently no life of its own. and The soul realm that is unseen but has the capability to receive both darkness and light.

It is the presence of the soul that makes the physical visible for though it light is passed on to the physical realm to emit and make it visible.

It is through this realm that the spirit realm passes life-containing light to the physical body to give it life.

This is the realm where the biochemicals operate in. It is the realm of physiological light.

The combination or balance of physiological light in this realm determines what happens in the physical bodily realm. It also determines what the physical body can receive from the spirit.

The spirit cannot pass light directly to the physical body, which will be destroyed by any direct contact. It is the light fields from the soul in the physical body that the spirit operates through.

Any deficiency in light fields is automatically occupied by darkness to enable the body operate as long as it has enough light to at least be existent.

In all these realms there is the presence of water. The manual tells us the word of our maker from which we are coded is also water even as it is light i.e. unseen water

This is the general basic principle of life. To understand all this and to do all that is necessary to ensure the soul can receive as much light fields as possible is to be empowered to live to the fullest.

We have no life in ourselves and therefore have none to pass on. We receive life from our maker. Only what he does has life for one cannot give what one does not have.

We have also shown ourselves to be totally irresponsible. We have been irresponsible with the little we can do. No one is going to give us any more. In fact our abilities will soon be removed as nature begins its self-repair system of removing every dangerous elements in its composition as coded.

The reason our inventions hurt is because they have no spirit content on their own, they are existing physical materials that we merge together. They have no living souls. They are not from nothing but a manipulation of things already in existence in the physical realm that the spirit of life has backed away from.

The Hebrew mathematical symbols can only operate in this realm as it is the realm of experimentation meant for knowledge only, to enable us understand the code of nature and the ways of our maker so we are careful not to violate his laws.

The human has only been given and can only effectively operate in a limited realm

The manual tells us the first man was given this realm to operate in as he named the various animals. The animals were already in existence. They already had life. They were already hydrated.

Humans were consequently coded to be assistants in innovation not the drivers. The maker will do the heavy lifting of providing life, hydration, processes and systems. All we are to do is maintain the system. That is the reason for the understanding we are given. To enable us maintain and appreciate the system

We have gone beyond our capability in our innovation, what was just for understanding we have stretched beyond the extent of its ability. Consequently the end products were not meant to be used as part of the actual living process.

Our maker in his own time will bring forth the real computers and other products that will actually have life and flow with nature.

Until then we are stuck with what we have unleashed.

This book and others I have written are the grace and mercy of our maker extended to us to enable survive in the corrupted system we have unleashed upon ourselves.

These books contain information to help us survive by making corrective step in our use of the tools we have come up with.

We must also heed the warning given to us by nature in things like global warming to let us know we have gone beyond the boundary so we can retrace our steps back from the brink and remain content with things within the atmosphere of the earth where the birds we are given jurisdiction over operate.

Airplanes carry us to and fro upon the earth. That is the boundary. The outer space is the place where control over us is exercised. We have no jurisdiction there except under the direct control of our maker who alone controls outer space.

How does this help us with staying hydrated
Now we know we cannot take things or granted. There is a limit to the amount of violation our bodies and indeed nature can tolerate before the self-repair system that is unleashed to battle our activities claims us as casualties.

It is not a struggle we can win. Nature will self repair and take us out to self-preserve. Our body's self-repair system can become overwhelmed.

Water is critical for us and dehydration is something we cannot afford to ignore as computer users.

Our bodies will never adjust to the dangers of dehydration and toxic poisoning inherent in computer use. We must put in preventive measures and adhere to them to survive in the environment we have unleashed upon ourselves.

When we understand our limits that the computer has no life or ability to help us control ourselves, then we know we cannot use it as a crutch or nanny to help us correct our behavior as many of us are doing today.

It is not the answer to everything and it must be used as a complementary tool to aid actual human activity and not to replace human activity.

We must take steps to ensure the violations of our coded way of being inherent in computer use do not destroy us.

One of the most important things as computer users we need to do for survival is to stay hydrated, as the computer cannot do that for us. We must adopt good lifestyle choices that ensure we are not overwhelmed when in the computer use environment.

The computer needs us to control it as we need our maker to control us and help us achieve success.

Let us begin our turnaround by getting the most basic things corrected by making an effort to remain properly hydrated at all times.

Note To The Reader:

About the author:

Adetutu Ijose, is a technology and accounting professional with over 25 years of intensive computer use exposure who suffered life threatening computer related health conditions the doctors could neither diagnose not treat.

In desperation and with a good knowledge of codes and how they work, she studied the human computer user manual we call the Bible until she was able to understand why and how the computer hurts our body's system as well as the preventive and repair kits placed in nature by our maker.

She also began to realize that many issues not normally attributable to computer use were actually due to or exacerbated by computer use.

One of those issues is the issue of dehydration, a condition many computer users are not aware they are at the risk of though they feel thirsty more that usual when using the computer or computer devices.

They just do not associate their thirst with dehydration and all its attendant consequences though they suffer these consequences.

That is because the dehydration is coupled with inherent neurotransmitter depletions.

Adetutu Ijose seeks in this book to bring this fact to everybody's attention in a bid to help computer users achieve and maintain a goo quality of life since computers are here to stay and are indispensable in today's world.

Because our modern lifestyle of heavy computer use is not going to change anytime soon, she realized that it was important to make the information she had public in a bid to help everyone.

She is now passing on her understanding about computer use induced issues through her many books, other writings and speaking activities so others can receive help.

Adetutu Ijose is a speaker on the subject of computer use induced health conditions. She is also a contributor to several online article websites and blogs including content sites Yahoo Contributor Network and examiner.com. She has also been interviewed on radio. She in addition became ordained as an Evangelist in 2008.

To schedule a speaking or consulting engagement, interview, so on with the author, please contact Adetutu Ijose at http://www.foodsthathealdaily.com.

For Adetutu Ijose's online press kit or for press releases and other media matters and inquiries, please go to http://lessosilearnedthehardway.com/AdetutuIjoseMediaPre ssKit.aspx

Discover other titles by Adetutu Ijose to help you better understand responsible computer use and how computer use affect us all as well as what we need to do to prevent and manage these issues at www.foodsthathealydaily.com, www.amazon.com and other online stores. Ebook versions of this and other books by Adetutu Ijose are available at amazon.com, Barnes and Nobles, Smashword.com and other ebook stores. A complete list is provided below.

Email Adetutu Ijose at adetutuijose@gmail.com or computerblessings@gmail.com

Connect with Adetutu Ijose Online:
Facebook: http://www.facebook.com/home.php

Read Adetutu Ijose's blogs at
http://lessonsilearnedthehardway.blogspot.com/ and
http://adetutuijose.wordpress.com/ and
http://www.foodsthathealdaily.com/Pages/Articlesandblogs.aspx

Computer Use Induced Health Conditions related books by Adetutu Ijose as at the time of writing are:

1)   *Lessons I Learned the Hard Way: How to Identify, Minimize, Treat and Manage Computer Related Health Condition*

2)   *Computer Related Health Condition: Understanding the Human Computer*

3)   *Healing Juicing Smoothie and Milk Shake Recipes: Juices, Smoothies and Milk Shakes that Help the Body Achieve its Self Healing Process*

4)   *Healing Meals Recipe: Meals that Help the Body Achieve its Self Healing Process*

5)   *Cyber Bullying: How and Why Bullies operate*

6)   *Global Epidemic: The Human Abuse of the Computer*

7)   *Computer Use Addiction and Withdrawal Syndromes: What You Need to Know*

8)   *Teenage and Adult Texting Addictions: What You Need to Know*

9)   *Allergies, Asthma and Computer Use: The Contributory Effects of Computer Use to Allergies and Asthma Trends*

10)   *Computer Use Induced Stress: What You Need to Know*

11)   *The Health effect of Video Games: What You Need to Know*

12)   *Eyes, Vision and Computer Use: How You can Protect Yourself From Technology Use Induced Harm*

13)   *Obesity and Computer Use: What You Need to Know*

14)   *Water, Dehydration and Computer Use: Learn How to Protect Yourself*

For other titles published after this book – Water, Dehydration and Computer Use, please go to amazon.com and other online stores or visit my website www.foodsthathealdaily.com Ebook versions are also available for kindle, ipad, kobo, sony, nook, smashwords.com and other ebook readers

References

1-1 The United States Geological Survey USGS) article on "The water within you" http://ga.water.usgs.gov/edu/propertyyou.html

3-1 Better Health Channel BHC), a service fully funded by the State Government of Victoria (Australi) article on water http://www.betterhealth.vic.gov.au/bhcv2/bhcarticles.nsf/pages/Water_a_vital_nutrient

4-1 Dr. Larry K Wan article on computer vision syndrome t http://www.allaboutvision.com/cvs/faqs.htm.

INDEX

L

Life, 5, 6, 9, 10, 11, 12, 26, 32, 34, 36, 42, 50, 53, 56, 57, 58, 59, 60, 67, 68, 69, 72

Light, 7, 10, 11, 12, 15, 17, 18, 22, 23, 24, 26, 27, 28, 30, 31, 32, 35, 36, 37, 38, 40, 41, 44, 45, 51, 52, 53, 56, 57, 60, 61, 63, 65, 66, 67, 68

M

Maker, 33, 34, 36, 44, 45, 46, 48, 50, 53, 54, 55, 56, 57, 61, 62, 63, 64, 65, 66, 67, 68, 69, 70, 71, 72

Manual, 5, 10, 11, 12, 32, 36, 40, 44, 49, 53, 60, 61, 62, 63, 65, 67, 68, 69, 72

Mathematical, 45, 51, 61, 69

Medical, 5, 6, 53

Medicated, 6, 7, 19

Medication, 6, 18, 19, 20, 29

Men, 13, 14, 26

Mental, 19, 25, 37, 66

Misdiagnosis, 19, 20, 31

Moisture, 9, 10, 12, 21, 22, 23, 24, 29, 32, 39, 44

Muscles, 15, 26, 40

N

Natural, 6, 7, 10, 19, 21, 26, 28, 36, 37, 40, 42, 47, 50, 54,

Nature, 5, 23, 32, 33, 34, 40, 44, 46, 47, 49, 52, 53, 54, 55, 56, 57, 68, 69, 70, 72

Natures mist, 27, 36, 39

Nerves, 15, 24, 35

Neurotransmitters, 22, 24, 25, 26, 33, 35, 36, 50, 61

O

Organ, 24, 25, 28

Organs, 15, 31, 40

P

People, 13, 14, 18,19, 25, 27, 36, 37, 42, 43, 51, 58, 59, 60, 61, 62, 65, 66
PH, 27, 28, 29, 35, 36
Pigmentation, 37, 65, 66, 67
Pigmented, 32, 36, 37

R

Realm, 57, 60, 67, 68, 69
Receptors, 21, 29, 35
Repair, 53, 54, 63, 70
Resources, 25, 30, 54

S

Science, 5, 9, 28, 50, 51, 53, 58, 61, 62, 65
Scriptures, 5, 10, 53, 44, 60, 61, 62
Self destruction, 34, 46, 64, 66
Skin, 10, 14, 21, 26, 27, 29, 35, 36, 37, 39, 41
Soda, 18, 25, 29, 38, 39
Software, 34, 53, 54
Solution, 5, 36, 55, 57, 65, 66
Solutions, 5, 6, 19, 29, 36, 47
Stress, 6, 24, 30, 75
Sun, 7, 19, 26, 32, 34, 35, 37, 40, 53
Sunlight, 11, 23, 24, 32, 33, 36, 37, 38
System, 5, 7, 10, 21, 22, 25, 28, 32, 22, 34, 38, 41, 45, 46, 48, 50, 51, 52, 53, 54, 65, 68, 69, 70, 72

T

Toxic, 17, 23, 26, 30, 40, 63, 64, 71
Toxins, 18, 22, 23, 31, 39, 40

U

Urine, 13, 14, 17, 18, 31

W